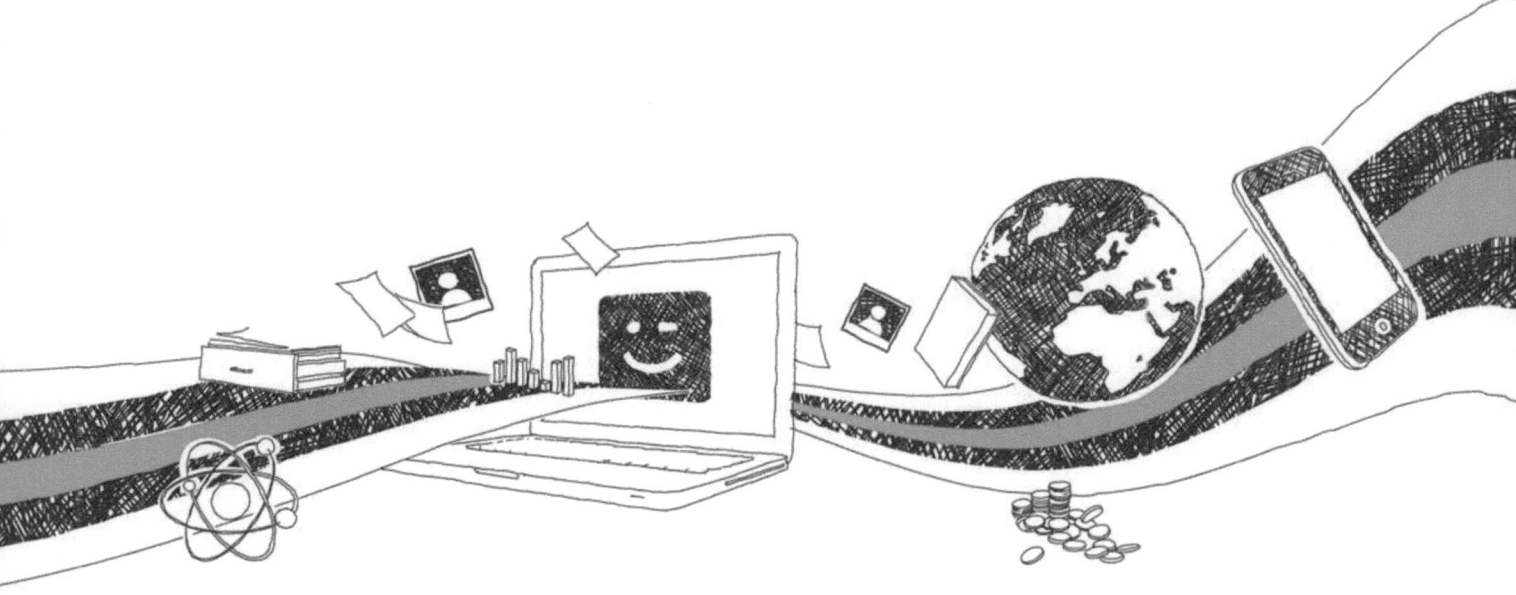
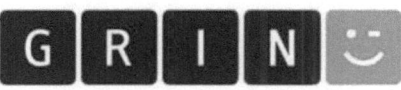

Darius Henatsch

Placental-Uterine Immunological Crosstalk

The Way the Prenatal Child Modulates the Maternal Immune Response to Prevent Its Own Rejection

GRIN Publishing

Bibliographic information published by the German National Library:

The German National Library lists this publication in the National Bibliography; detailed bibliographic data are available on the Internet at http://dnb.dnb.de .

Imprint:

Copyright © 2007 GRIN Verlag GmbH
Print and binding: Books on Demand GmbH, Norderstedt Germany
ISBN: 978-3-640-90929-2

This book at GRIN:

http://www.grin.com/en/e-book/134744/placental-uterine-immunological-crosstalk

GRIN - Your knowledge has value

Since its foundation in 1998, GRIN has specialized in publishing academic texts by students, college teachers and other academics as e-book and printed book. The website www.grin.com is an ideal platform for presenting term papers, final papers, scientific essays, dissertations and specialist books.

Visit us on the internet:

http://www.grin.com/

http://www.facebook.com/grincom

http://www.twitter.com/grin_com

Placental-Uterine Immunological Crosstalk

The Way, the Prenatal Child Modulates the Maternal Immune

Response to Prevent Its Own Rejection.

Caspar Darius Henatsch
Molecular Life Science
Maastricht University (tUL)

Contents

Abbreviations	
Ag	antigen
APC	antigen presenting cell
APRIL	a proliferation-inducing factor
BAFF	B cell-activating factor belonging to the TNF family
CD	cluster of differentiation
CSF	colony stimulating factor
CTL	cytotoxic T lymphocyte
EVT	extra villous trophoblasts
GM	granulocyte-macrophage
GnRH	gonadotropin releasing hormone
hCG	human chorionic gonadotropin
HLA	human leukocyte antigen
IFN	interferon
IL	interleukin
ILT	Ig-like transcript
ITIM	immunoreceptor tyrosine based inhibition motifs
ITAM	immunoreceptor tyrosine based activation motifs
KIR	killer cell Ig-like receptor
NK cell	natural killer cell
MHC	histocompatibility complex
PBMC	peripheral blood mononuclear cell
PGE	Prostaglandin
RT-PCR	reverse transcription-polymerase chain reaction
TCR	T cell receptor
TGF	transforming growth factor
Th	T helper
TNF	tumour-necrosis factor
Treg cell	regulatory Tcell
uNK cell	uterine NK cell

Table 1: List of abbreviations.

1. Introduction

Approximate 100 million years ago an important evolutionary event occurred, the diversification of the stem of eutherian (placental) mammals.[3,4] In this transition from oviparity to viviparity, the mammalian success mainly depended on the simultaneous forming of a transient and omnipotent organ: The placenta.[5,6]

Viviparity gave rise to new advantages like the embryonic development in a safe inter-maternal environment as well as an advanced system in nutrient and waste-product exchange, compared to yolk-sac nutrition.[7]

For the intense placental-uterine fusion with a warranty of effectual anastomosis concerning the necessary embryonic supply, a fine-tuned and high coordinated trophoblast cell invasion of the uterine tissues and the uterine spiral arterial walls is required.[6,8] This event of placentation and thus the infiltration of extra villous trophoblasts (EVT) in the decidua, the maternal uterine membrane, equals the concept of transplantation.[9] The placenta is, as well as the embryo, a semi-allograft, possessing antigens from both, maternal and paternal origin. The anticipation for the penetration of genetic differing material is the immediate initiation of a broad immune response, which is not true in case of the placenta. So an immunological unique placental-uterine crosstalk is established in the uterine side of EVT exposure. Humans have haemochorial placentae, marked by extensive invasion of trophoblasts, which define the boundary between mother and fetus. These cells have unique patterns of gene expression and develop independently from embryonic tissue.[7]

The main issue of this paper is the question how the placenta, in particular placental trophoblast cells, prevent a maternal allograft immune rejection by modulating the immune response in the uterine side of implantation.

The attempt is done to give insights about special immunological interactions at the placental-uterine side of implantation that makes the fascinating event of pregnancy possible.

Of main interest are interactions between trophoblast human leukocyte antigens (HLAs), natural killer (NK) cells as well as T lymphocytes, in questions of state of the art literature. Although a broad introduction is given to the development of the embryo until nidation; how the uterus is made up during implantation and the mechanisms of placentation.

2. The Uterus

The uterus can be seen as the major female reproduction organ, the side where the embryo and fetus sojourns during the time of pregnancy.

2.1 Anatomy and Alteration in the Cycle

The endometrium, the outermost part of the epithelial layer of the uterus, pulls apart and reconstructs every 28 days in the normal menstrual cycle in women of child-bearing age.

The cycle begins with a proliferative phase in terms of refashioning of the endometrium, whereas a 9 day period antecedent ovulation marks strongly growths in size of the epithelial layer which gets richly vascularized as well as strongly infiltrated by NK cells. The moment of ovulation is followed by a 14-day secretory phase, in which NK cells proliferate and differentiate to create a site best attractive for embryonic implantation.[3] The short period of time where implantation is possible due to unique, hormone affected endometrial modulation is called the *implantation window*. It is regulated by the cyclic secretion of 17β-estradiol and progesterone, responsible for the regulation of growth factors, cytokines and adhesion molecules that alter the endometrial surface to open the implantation window by creating the best possible epithelial environment for placental trophoblast ingrowths. The window is closed after several days by amongst others fibronectin.[8] Also, if no fertilization and implantation takes place, NK cells die and the five-day period of menstruation, the flaking of the endometrial layer, occurs.[3]

2.2 Special Make-up during Embryonic Nidation

The ´decidual reaction` is a cellular and vascular change occurring to the endometrium in response to embryonic implantation.[8] For an adequate oxygen and nutrition supply of the embryo the endometrium has to remodel into the decidua, a much-changed tissue highly nerved by blood vessels.[3] This process is initiated perpetual the opening of the implantation window during the menstruation cycle whereas decidualisation accumulates glycogen and lipids in epithelial cells causing their typical enlargement and pail-staining appearance. The exact function of the decidua stays vague but it can be adopt that besides the facilitation of implantation it plays a main role in restraining and controlling the massive trophoblast invasion.[8]

3. The Placenta

The placenta forms an organ between embryo/fetus and the uterus of the mother during pregnancy, ensuring adequate exchange of oxygen, nutrients and waste products and is responsible for remodeling processes of the uterine immune cell population and the maternal uterine arteries.[6,8]

3.1 From Fertilization to Nidation

Fertilization takes place in the ampulla of the oviduct, a region close to the ovary, by penetration of the spermatozoa through the zona pellicula of the ovulated oocyte: The zygote is formed with a diploid complement of chromosomes.

In the next 24 hours the zygote is pushed by cilia of the oviduct down in direction of the uterus and undergoes mitotic cell division known as cleavage, whereas new daughter cells, the blastomeres, are formed. By day 4 the embryo consists of 32 cells and is called morula. (Figure 2) Blastomeres in the center of the morula give rise to the inner cell mass, whereas cells of the periphery develop into the outer cell mass. The inner cell mass will further transfer into the embryo proper called the embryoblast. The outer cell mass, by primary forming the source of the chorion, the embryonic portion of the placenta, is called trophoblast (trophectoderm). The morula begins to absorb fluid, which shapes a cavity called the blastocyst cavity.

The trophoblast cells are now arranged in a thin outer cell layer around the blastocyst cavity and the embryoblast forms a compact mass at one side of the cavity, the embryonic pole, and is called the blastocyst.

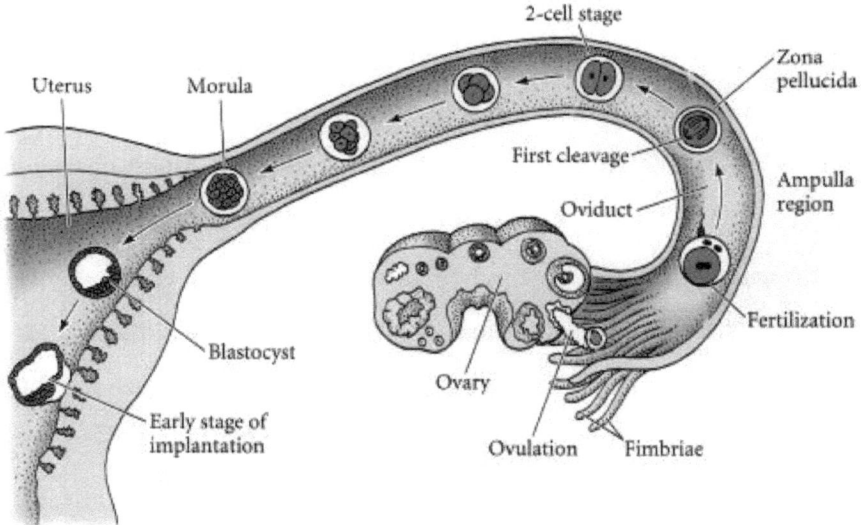

Figure 2: Development of a human embryo; from feritlization to implantation.[10]

The zona pellicula, which surrounds the blastocyst, prevents the embryo form adhering to the oviduct walls. Between day 3 and 4, the morula reaches the uterus and the blastocyst gets tightly bound to the uterine lining, by hatching from the zona pellicula. After that initial binding process, several adhesion systems ensure and coordinate a successful binding to the uterine wall.[11,12] After the zona pellicula is lost and the binding took place, the blastocyst sinks beneath the endometrial surface.[8]

3.2 Implantation and Placentation

The route of placentation begins after the blastocyst has implanted into the uterine epithelium and the process of differentiation into inter-, and extra-embryonic tissue is achieved.[13] Immediately after attachment, rapid proliferation of the trophoblast cell layer of the blastocyst takes place and differentiates into an inner cytotrophoblastic layer and an outer multinucleated syncytiotrophoblastic mass.[8]

At day 13 to 14 of pregnancy cytotrophoblast cells penetrate through the outer embryonic shell, which is composed of syncytiotrophoblasts, begin the invasion of the uterine stroma and give rise to the cell line of extravillous cytotrophoblasts and villous cytotrophoblast. (Figure 3)[8,13]

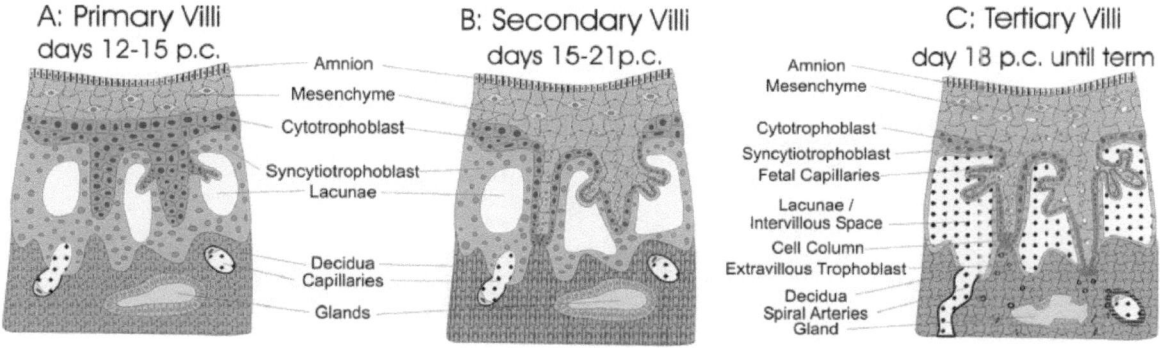

Figure 3: Growth of placental villi. A: Ingrowths of cytotrophoblasts into the syncitiotrophoblast cell layer leads to formation of primary villi. B: Secondary villi are formed by mesnchyme migration. C: Remodeling of maternal spiral arteries occurred and tertiary villi are formed.[13]

Former function in two ways: locating and surrounding of the spiral arteries (uterine arterial circulation) and the mediation of an adaptive maternal response to the implantation of the embryo. This happens due to endocrine communication, inducing the onset of a successful pregnancy.

EVTs that proliferate inside the decidual spiral arteries are named ´endovascular trophoblasts` and primary prevent maternal blood-flow into the developing intervillous space until the placental disc has formed. Afterwards they replace the muscularized wall of the spiral arteries to ensure a sufficient blood flow to the intervillous space, which is, additively stimulated by angiogenic and vasodilator signals.[3,6,8,13]

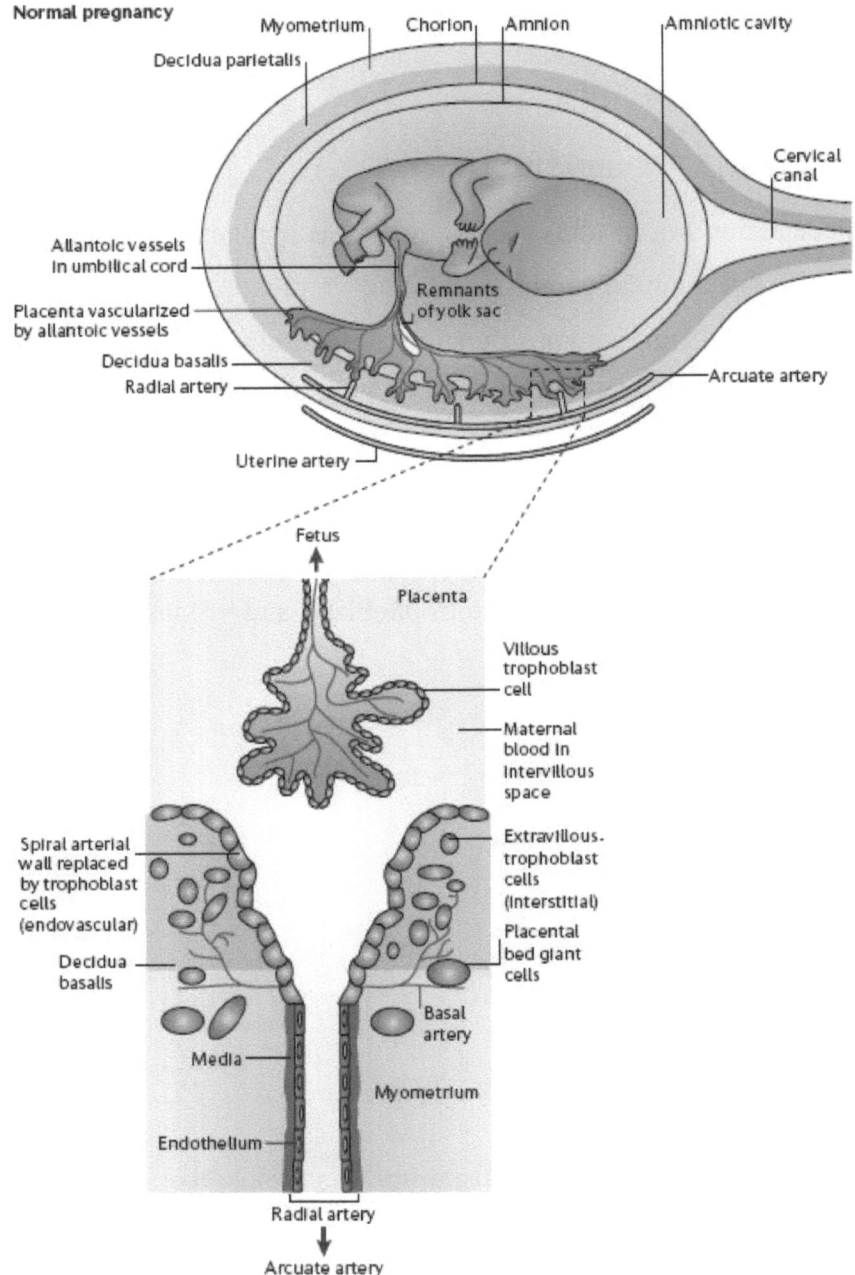

Figure 4: Placentation in a normal pregnancy.[7]

Maternal blood vessels create large, flaccid ducts to comply the great demand of blood from the fetus, especially from the developing fetal brain that consumes nearly 60% of nutritional needs in the third trimester, which explains the extra deep infiltration in humans.[3,6,7]

Another subpopulation of extravillous trophoblasts, the interstitial trophoblasts, transform into multinucleated placental bed giant cells and migrate deep into the decidua. Villous cytotrophoblast do not migrate but give rise to the choronic villi by fusing with the outer shell, the syncytiotrophoblast, and by forming the villous core, which is later on (third week of gestation) filled by mesenchyme.[8] Feto-placental blood vessels are formed in the extra-embryonic mesenchyme, by vasculogenesis of embryonic mesoderm. This tissue penetrates the more proximal layer of cytotrophoblast, giving rise to the 'tertiary choronic villi`, the forerunners of the gas-exchanging choronic villi. Later on latter will form the mature villous tree that is covered by the 'vasculo-syncytial membrane` (syncytiotrophoblast), proximal to the umbilical arteries as a border between maternal and fetal blood.[13,14] It is important to distinguish between the floating villi that are suspended within the intervillous space and the anchoring villi, attached to the maternal decidua.[14] Serious clinical conditions arise if trophoblasts invasion not proceed far enough or when the transformation of maternal vessels is incomplete. The result is an inadequate blood flow later on in pregnancy, the primary defect in Pre-eclampsia and intrauterine growth retardation (IUGR).[6]

3.3 Function

The placenta shows a fascinating ability to differentiate in a short period of time from the trophectoderm into a full-fledged multifunctional organ.[5] It has to ensure adequate nutrition of the developing embryo and fetus, to take over parts of hormonal pregnancy control and forms a unique immunological barrier between the maternal and fetal circulation.

3.3.1 Nutrition

The placenta is a haemochorial villous organ, creating direct contact between maternal blood and placental trophoblasts at the site where oxygen, nutrition and waste-product exchange takes place.[8] During the process of placentation a close contact between the interface of the maternal and fetal circulatory systems must be established to ensure this exchange in a sufficient manner. Herein a very important fact is that no direct contact of blood evolves between uterine blood vessels and fetal blood.[14] For the continuous supply of the developing fetus, maternal blood needs efficient access to the layer of multinucleated syncytiotrophoblast, which is made possible by the remodeling of maternal spiral arteries in the uterus by invasive mononucleated trophoblasts (discussed earlier).[5]

The placenta ensures transport of oxygen, water, carbohydrates, lipids, vitamins, minerals and other nutrients to the fetus, while removing carbon dioxide and other waste products.[8]

3.3.2 The Placenta as a Hormonal Organ

The placenta is a temporally hormonal organ, secreting hormones and cytokines, indispensable for the normal maturation and protection of the developing fetus, amongst others progesterone, estrogens (like oestrone, oestradiol and oestriol), human chorionic gonadotrophin (hCG), as well as many cytokines and chemokines.[5,8] Progesterone is very important for the inhibition of uterine contractions, whereas estrogens act as growth hormones on maternal reproductive organs like breast, uterus, cervix and vagina.[8] The glucoprotein hormone hCG is produced and secreted at high amounts by the syncytiotrophoblasts and is positively regulated by the gonadotropin releasing hormone (GnRH). It is responsible for the fusion of cytotrophoblasts and the differentiation of villous trophoblasts.[5,8]

Progesterone and prostaglandins are also immunosuppressants, reducing maternal immune reactions. Trophoblasts produce amongst others the chemokines CXCL12 and the stromal cell factor-1, which are able to attract immune cells of the innate immune system and are in that way responsible for a shift from acquired to innate immunity in the uterus, important for successful implantation of the conceptus.[2]

3.3.3 Barrier between Fetal and Maternal Circulation

The placenta as an intermediary organ between fetus and maternal tissue assures the complete separation of both circulation systems, to prevent a maternal immunological reaction against, and rejection of, the fetus as a semi-allograft. Besides this the placenta is a barrier not only for xenobiotics but also for a brought rage of bacteria and viruses, found in maternal blood. Important is that this function is related to a lot but not all substances and microorganisms.[8]

4. Immunological Uterine-Placental Crosstalk

In non-pathological pregnancies a balance is achieved between fetal and maternal cells with a definitive boundary line demarcating their respective territories, wherein neither excessive rejection nor an immoderate nidation takes place. This process needs fine-tuned cellular interactions in areas around the borderline. [6]

4.1 Immunologic Reaction to Foreign, Allogeneic Tissue

The fetus can be seen as an allogeneic graft, carrying beside maternal antigens (Ags) also paternal Ags, genetically disparate from maternal tissue.[15,16] Under normal circumstances the placenta as fetal tissue would be recognized as foreign, producing an excessive production of graft-attacking antibodies as well as stimulating a massive cytotoxic T lymphocytes (CTL) response, resulting in the rejection of the fetus, similar to what is seen in tissue and organ transplantations.[7,16] So the gene expression pattern of the placenta must somehow be different from that of the embryo and fetus.

4.2 Maternal Cells Involved in Direct Interactions

Immunological cells abundant in site of the uterus are a population of infiltrating CD (cluster of differentiation) 45[+] leukocytes which is, during times of decidualization, composed for approximate 70 per cent (50-90%) of CD56 [bright] NK cells, macrophages and some T-lymphocytes, whereas B cells are nearly absent.[2,3,6,7,9]

One can distinguish between two NK cell types, CD56[bright] (high CD56 expression) and CD56[dim] (low CD56 expression). Former are specialized in cytokine expression, with transcription levels three fold higher in at least 200 different genes, compared to CD56[dim], which are specialized in cytolysis.[3,33] If the uterine NK subpopulation is derived from peripheral precursor cells of arises in situ is not known.[3,14] Another difference in decidual and peripheral cell population is seen in the T cell population. Some decidual T cells express the gamma delta positive T cell receptor (TCR $\gamma\delta^+$), rarely found in the peripheral population (~5%), which are expected to form a first-line defends because they can be found more frequent in epithelial tissues. $\gamma\delta$ T cells do not recognize major histocompatibility complex (MHC) associated peptide antigens but seem to be able to spot antigens directly.[14,17] Other uterine T cells are the CD4[+] CD25[bright] regulatory T (Treg) cells, which are involved in suppression of an aggressive allogeneic response against the fetus.

Also a shift of pro-inflammatory T helper (Th) 2 cytokines to anti-inflammatory Th1 cytokines can be seen.[2,15] There is a clear difference in the uterine T cell response in the pregnant and non-pregnant endometrium. This response is the same like in other tissues in the non-pregnant state, seen for example in a rapid production of granulomas after endometrial bacterial infections.[7]

Furthermore there is a rare NKT cell type found in the uterine decidua, bearing both, receptor characteristics of NKs and T cells. Their importance in pregnancy in not clearly described but a subtype, the invariant NKT cells are able to bind to CD1d, a ligant that belongs to the non-classical MHC class I like molecules.[14]

4.3 NK Cell Receptor Interactions

NKs, cells of the innate immunity, circulate through the periphery, checking nucleated cells weather their self-MHC possesses a normal profile. These as well as the up-regulation of special surface molecules are signs of DNA damage or cell stress due to infection and transformation. Two receptor complexes are involved in this accurate process, the killer cell immunoglobulin-like receptor (KIR) and the inhibitory CD94-NKG2A complex. Another receptor of the NKs is the NKG2D that is activated by the ´stress-state` of the target cell.

Furthermore they have a heterogeneous arsenal of receptors, which let them respond to cytokines and microbial factors.[18,19] A distinctive NK cell type is found in the uterine mucosa, the $CD56^{bright}/CD16^-$ that can recognize the semi-allogeneic fetal trophoblast HLA-G, HLA-C and HLA-E due to the existence of a special set of receptors.[9] The expression of trophoblast MHC class I molecules seems to be not only directly responsible for inhibition of the cytolytic function of uNKs but also for an alteration of the uNK cytokine repertoire. Amongst others high productions of granulocyte-macrophage colony stimulating factor (GM-CSF), IFN-γ, colony stimulating factor (CST) 1 and tumour-necrosis factor (TNF) have been found, in combination with a high expression of receptors on invading trophoblasts. This leads to the expectation that uNKs have an important effect on EVT cell behavior.[6]

The ligand-receptor interactions could be proven by cytotoxicity assays using target cells transfected with class I molecules as well as by direct binding assays using soluble fusion proteins like KIR, Ig-like transcript (ILT) and CD94/NKG2.[9]

4.3.1 CD94/NKG2

Uterine NK cells express high levels of the inhibitory CD94/NKG2A receptor. Both, maternal cells and trophoblasts express the ligand, HLA-E. So this ligand receptor interaction with uNK cells prevents any uNK cell derived cell lyses in the vicinity.[6]

The CD94/NKG2 (C-type lectin like molecule) is a member of the C-type lectin superfamily and forms a heterodimer (CD94-NKG2) for binding with the non-classical HLA-E molecule. A division can be made into two CD94/NKG2 subtypes, the NKG2A and the NKG2C.[9]

NKG 2A

It could be shown by flow-cytometry measurements that nearly all decidual CD56^{bright} NKs express CD94/NKG2A at five times greater levels than blood NK cells. The majority (about 95 per cent) of these cells also show a high binding affinity to the soluble HLA-E tetrameric complex.

Stimulation of this receptor subtype, which is the case after contact with trophoblasts of the semi allograft, leads to an inhibitory signal, regarding to the NK cell induced cell-lyses.

The CD94/NKG2A complex is coupled to intracellular immunoreceptor tyrosine based inhibition motifs (ITIMs) that are responsible for the induction of the inhibitory signal transduction. (Figure 5)[7,9]

NKG 2C

The NKG2C receptor subtype produces, contrary to NKG2A, an activating signal when ligand-stimulated. It contains no intracellular ITIMs but is associated with the signal molecule DAP-12, which contains immunoreceptor tyrosine based activation motifs (ITAMs). (Figure 5)

The affinity of NKG2C to HLA-E is significantly lower than for NKG2A, resulting in a net inhibition of cell-lyses activity of uNKs, when stimulated. Both receptor subtypes generate the highest binding-affinity to HLA-E when the leading sequence of HLA-G is additively bound in its binding groove.[6,9,20]

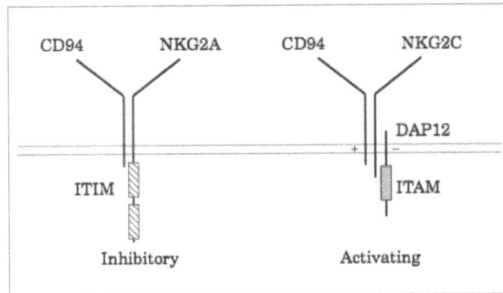

Figure 5: Inhibitory CD94/NKG2A and activating CD94/NKG2C complex.[9]

UNK cells also express an activating CD94/NKG2C receptor that can only bind the HLA-E-HLA-G leader sequence complex with an affinity high enough to trigger a cell response. This arises the opportunity for uNK cells to respond *in utero* differently to trophoblast HLA-E compared to other surrounding HLA-E positive but HLA-G negative maternal cells. In that way HLA-G can influence and alter the maternal response being presented by HLA-E even when the fetus is HLA-G null homozygote because only the leader peptide is need to be translated.[6]

4.3.2 KIR (killer cell Ig-like receptor)

In pregnant women, a greater proportion of uNKs express members of the KIR multi-gene family, specific for HLA-C cells than peripheral blood NK cells. The CD56^{bright} NK cell subpopulation in the periphery does not express KIRs. This is not the case in CD56^{bright} uNKs, what leads to the expectation that this special subset expression pattern is induced *in utero*.

Women express KIRs for a wide range of HLA-Cs that are polymorphic, including both groups of HLA-C alleles, maternal as well as paternal. In consequence different combinations of paternal non-self fetal HLA-C and maternal uNK cell expressed KIRs are found in different pregnancies. The randomized matching of ligant and receptor could be an influence for pathological syndromes like Pre-eclampsia or even pregnancy failure.[6]

The KIR locus consists of 7-15 closely packed genes, giving rise to numerous haplotypes, differing in both, gene content and allele combination. Two groups, A and B, are formed. The simpler group, group A haplotype, contains mainly genes for inhibitory receptors, whereas the more complicated group of B haplotype contains genes for activating ones.

The disease Pre-eclampsia more often refers to women homozygote for the A haplotype (AA) than to women heterozygote (AB) of B homozygote (BB).[3]

The matching of KIR and HLA-C allotypes are important in pregnancies. HLA-C forms two groups; the C1 and C2 group. Former is the ligant for the inhibitory KIR2DL2 and KIR2DL3 with asparagine at position 80, whereas the C2 group forms the ligant for the activating

KIR2DS1 and the inhibitory KIR2DL1 with lysine at position 80. The C2 group shows a higher binding affinity than the C1 one.

Pre-eclampsia here more often refers to homozygote AA women with homozygote C2 (C2C2) or heterozygote (C1C2) embryos. The reason therefore is that the C2 group ligants bind tightly to their inhibitory KIR receptor counterpart.[3,7]

This shows the importance of KIR-HLA-C interaction between uterine NK cells and extravillous trophoblasts for an effective spiral artery remodeling process to ensure an adequacy in embryonic and fetal blood supply.

The KIR receptor is encoded by 10 different genes and consists of two (KIR2D) or three (KIR3D) extra-cellular domains, with varying, short (S) or long (L) tails. KIR2D predominantly interacts with HLA-C. Like the CD94/NKG2 receptor, KIR also has different subtypes, leading to different intercellular pathways.[9,19]

KIR2/3DL

The KIR2DL subtype can be compared to the NKG2A subtype, also coupled to the long tailed ITIM that exhibits an inhibitory signal when stimulated. (Figure 6)

KIR2/3DS

This receptor subtype, like NKG2C is coupled to DAP-12-ITAM, relaying an activating signal. (Figure 6)[9,19]

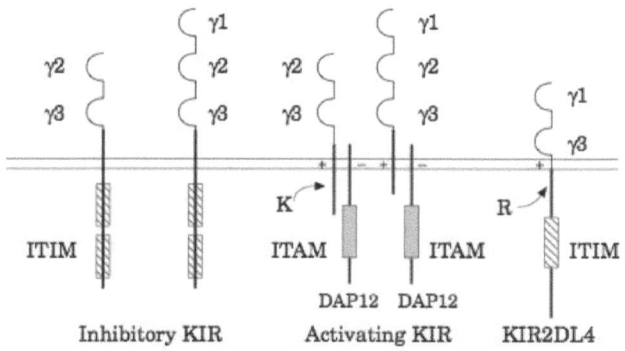

Figure 6: Structures of inhibiting and activating KIRs.[9]

KIR2DL4

This member of the KIR gene-family is evolutionary conserved and is expressed by all NK cells. KIR2DL4 receptor stimulation activates cytokine production and is not involved in cytotoxicity, whereas it is suggested that HLA-G is its ligant. The main cytokine produced by this stimulation is IFNγ.[6,19,20]

4.3.3 ILT (Ig-like transcript)

ILT can be found not only on NK cells but on a wide range of monocytes like B, and T cells, whereas ILT4 expression is more related to the myelomonocytic lineage.[9,21] The ILT family consist of at least eight different members but only ILT2 and ILT4 can bind HLA class I molecules, especially HLA-G.[9] Both ILTs have four tandem Ig-like extra-cellular domains, linked to intracellular ITIMs. It could be shown that ILT2 binds with the highest affinity to HLA-G1, resulting in a peripheral blood NK cell inhibition, not only leading to materno-fetal tolerance but also to the escape of tumor cells.[21]

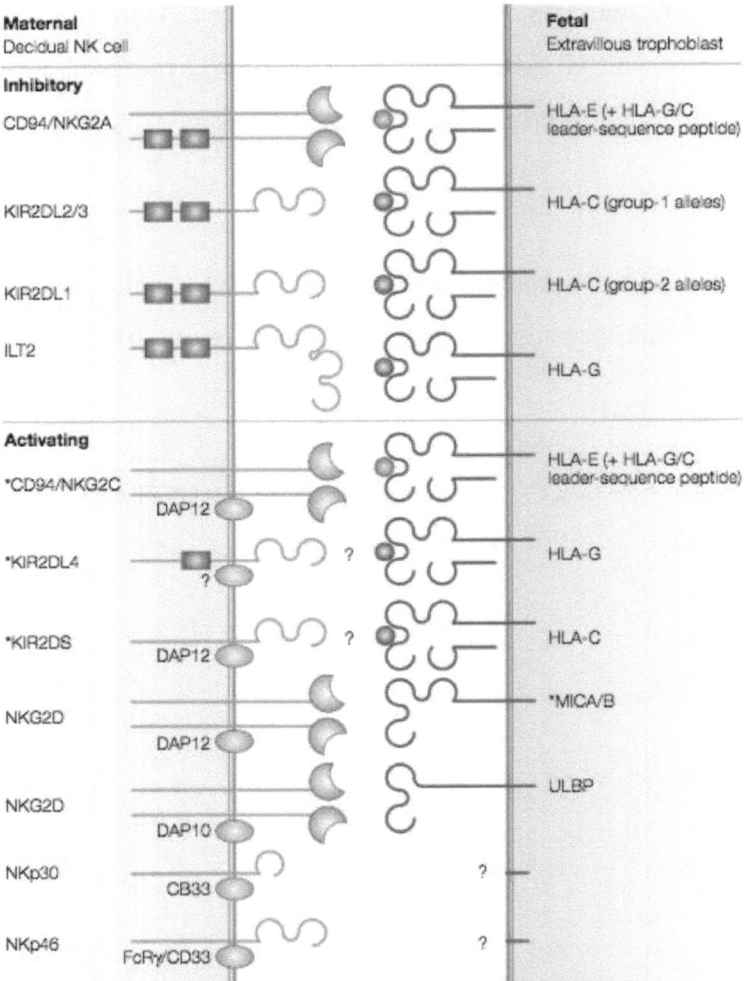

Figure 7: Receptor-ligant interaction between placental expressed HLAs and maternal uterine NK cells.[6]

5. Major Histocompatibility Complex (MHC) Expression on Placental Cells

Placental trophoblast cells show a special MHC expression pattern not found on other cells in the body, what gives them the opportunity of unique communication with cells of maternal origin.[16]

5.1 Human Leukocyte Antigens (HLAs)

Genes encoding human leukocyte antigens are clustered on chromosome 6p21 at the telomeric end of the HLA region. HLAs can be subdivided into class Ia, HLA-A, HLA-B, HLA-C, class Ib, HLA-F and HLA-G and class II, HLA-D antigens.[16,22]

Class Ia antigens can be found on the membrane on nearly every nucleus containing body cell, with a high expression on lymphocytes and macrophages. Class II antigens are just found on the cell membranes of antigen presenting cells (APCs), like B cells, activated T cells, macrophages, endothelial cells, Langerhans cells of the epidermis and spermatocytes.[22]

Just a few of the approximate 20-25 HLA class I antigens genes are transcribed and translated because many are pseudogenes or gene fragments. HLA class Ia antigens are much more polymorphic compared to HLA class Ib antigens. HLA-E has two, HLA-G five and HLA-F just one allele.[16]

Placental cells have an atypical MHC expression pattern, leading to the expectation that they function amongst others as special ligands for uterine immune cells, including T cells, NK cells and myelomonocytic cells.[7]

Normal cells of the human body express the MHC class I molecules HLA-A and HLA-B, important for antigen presentation to B, T cells and NK cells. NK cells of the innate immune system recognize to low or absent expression of MHC class I, which results in NK cell mediated killing of the target cells (invaders such as bacteria or virus infected cells).[14,23]

This is neither happening with the fetal-derived trophoblasts cells of the placental villi that do not at all express MHC class I nor to the deeply invasive extravillous cytotrophoblast, expressing only HLA-C and the non-classical HLA-E and HLA-G.[6,7,14]

5.2 Characteristics of Classical and Non-classical MHC Class I Molecules

Some features of the trophoblast class I molecules show that they do not function primarily in antigen presentation. HLA-C products exhibit polymorphism but have a relatively short half-life at the cell surface, which limits the efficiency in Ag presentation.

HLA-E and HLA-G show limited polymorphisms, which makes them inappropriate Ag-presenters, whereas in vitro studies demonstrated an opportunity of HLA-G to communicate with CD8$^+$ T cells, by binding a diverse set of antigenic peptides in its peptide-binding cleft.[14]

The trophoblast HLA expression pattern just includes, besides HLA class Ib antigens, HLA-C, but not A and B. The expression of the polymorphic HLA-C alone is more than enough for an allograft rejection reaction, which is not the case in successful pregnancies. So unique features of that mixed expression pattern must modulate the maternal immune response.[16]

5.3 Subgroups of Trophoblast HLA Class I Antigens

Trophoblast express only HLA-C as a class Ia antigen and besides HLA-G just the non-classical HLA class Ib antigen HLA-E.[16]

5.3.2 HLA-C

HLA-C exists in two different forms, the β_2m bound and the free heavy chain form, with an up-regulation stimulated by interferon (IFN) γ.[9]

Maternal decidual NK cells appear to have a higher HLA-C recognition pattern compared to those in the peripheral blood, by expressing the receptor KIR2D.[24]

The Maps GL183$^+$ and EB6$^+$ are specific for KIR2D receptors that bind the two groups of HLA-C allotypes. Using these Maps it could be found out that there are 50-80 per cent of CD56^{bright} decidual NK cells reactive with either or both Maps compared with 5-20 per cent of Map reactive NK cells of the periphery from the same pregnant woman. So there is an increased recognition of HLA-C of maternal uNK cells compared to those of the periphery.[9,24]

5.3.1 HLA-E

These molecules are only present on the cell surface and not like other HLA class I molecules as well in the ER (endoplasmatic reticulum).[9] HLA-E commonly presents antigenic peptides derived from the signal peptide sequence (leader sequence) of other MHC class I molecules.

Peptides destined for the cell surface are translated at the ribosome with a leader sequence at their N-terminus to enter the lumen of the ER through the pore formed by the Sec61 complex. The leader sequence is then enzymatically removed by signal peptidase and the peptide normally presented at the cell surface by MHC class I products.[14]

HLA-E has the ability to bind both HLA-G as well as HLA-C in its binding groove and may in that way present beside itself also these two other HLA class I molecules to uNK (uterine NK) cells. This gives uNK cells the possibility to ´sense` and react to HLA-G positive fetal trophoblasts.[9]

6. Special role of HLA-G

HLA-G is a specific MHC class 1b antigen with only few alleles compared to the other highly polymorphic HLA-A and HLA-B.[16] HLA-G expression is tissue/organ specific and/or conditional and is expressed, besides by extravillous trophoblasts, only by medullary epithelial cells of the thymus and activated monocytes. HLA-C and HLA-E are ubiquitously expressed.[3,16,25]

6.1 Unique HLA-G Features

HLA-G bears special functions in its appearance based on alternative splicing abilities forming, among four membrane-bound forms, three soluble isoforms (HLA-G1 to HLA-G7), shown by amongst others reverse transcription-polymerase chain reaction (RT-PCR) studies. Just two of the soluble forms, HLA-G5 and HLA-G6 play a role in pregnancy.[2,16,25,26] This unique feature is not seen in other class I antigens which are all membrane bound. HLA-G has eight exons encoding a signal peptide (exon 1), α1-3 domains (exon 2-4 respectively) a trans- membrane domain (exon 5) and an intracellular domain (exon 6 and 7). (Figure 8)

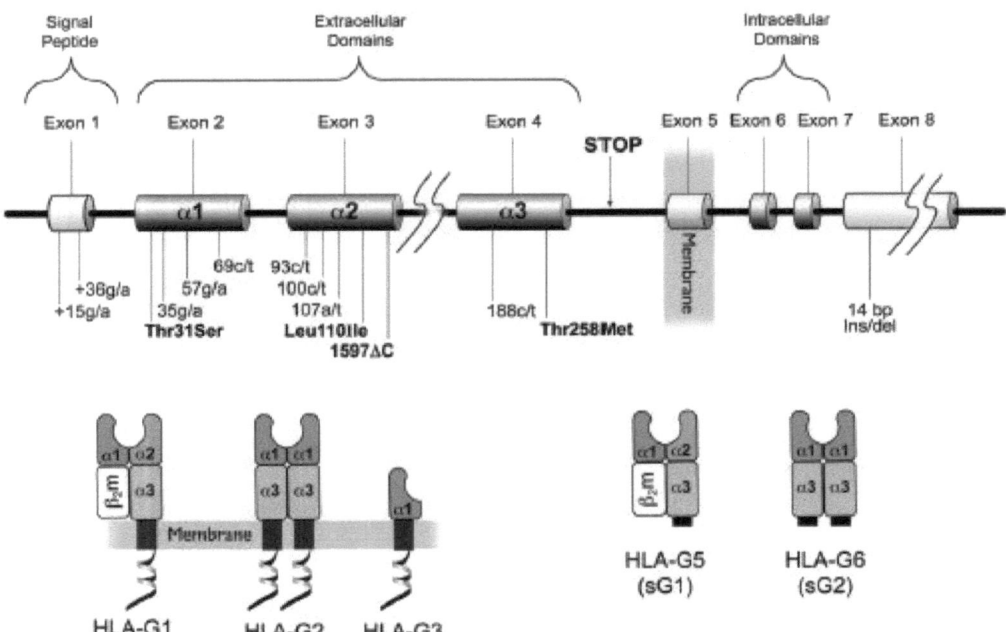

Figure 8: Alternative mRNA splicing results in several HLA-G proteins. Upper: 8 exons are transcribed to produce 7 different splicing variants, of which are three soluble forms. Lower: Three encoded membrane bound isoforms and two encoded soluble ones.[16]

By using special labeling techniques HLA-G2/G6 can be labeled by anti G2/G6 (26-2H11) showing that the expression of one or both of these isoforms is induced by migrating extravillous cytotrophoblasts as well as the soluble HLA-G5 (sG1), stained by anti G5 (1-2C3). (Figure 9)[16] The expression is further related to macrophages in choronic villi and endothelial cells lining fetal placental blood vessels.[27]

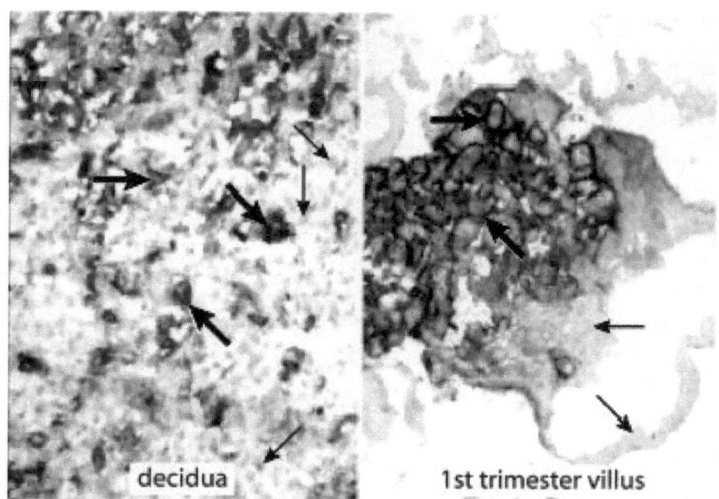

Figure 9: Labeling for HLA-G2/G6 and HLA-G5 during cytotrophoblast migration in the decidua. Left: first trimester decidua. Right: cytotrophoblast column.[16]

6.2 HLA-G Interactions with Maternal Cells

HLA-G was found to bind mainly to ILT receptors, more precisely to ILT2 and ILT4, which are expressed by T- and B-lymphocytes and mononuclear macrophages as well as by NK cells.[9,16,20,27,28] More precisely these receptor interactions are maintained via ILT2/CD85j, ILT4/CD85d and also by KIR2DL4/CD158d.[26] At the maternal-fetal interface, levels of the ILT receptor type high enough to be detectable, are found in macrophages rather then NK cells. There can still be a response of decidual NKs to HLA-G via ILT2, whereas this ligant-binding could not be proven for sure.[9] As mentioned earlier, besides the membrane bound variants, also two different soluble splicing variants of HLA-G exist.

6.2.1 T Cell Interactions

Soluble as well as membrane-bound HLA-G molecules have shown to be able to modulate cytokine release from human allogeneic peripheral mononuclear cells. APCs transfected with HLA-G1 are able to prevent CD4$^+$ T cell proliferation and turn them toward an immunosuppressive Th-2 cytokine producing lymphocyte phenotype rather than into the Th-1 one. That produces a milieu more favorable for pregnancy maintenance. A failure to achieve this preference of Th-2 cytokine producing T lymphocytes leads to unsuccessful pregnancies.[16,29] The amounts of Th-2 stimulating cytokines, like interleukin (IL) -3 and IL-4 rose in culture medium of a mHLA-G transfected B-lymphoblast cell line and peripheral blood mononuclear cells (PBMCs), whereas the amount of Th-1 stimulating cytokines, like TNF-α and INF-γ were significantly reduced.[25,30]

Studies of HLA-G1 transfected APC lines showed that these cells were able to induce the differentiation of CD4[+] T cells into suppressive CD4[+] T cells. The inhibition of activation, proliferation and differentiation of these cells reduce their maturation stimulation of CD8[+] T cells into cytotoxic T cells dramatically. HLA-G1 induces concentration and time of incubation dependent long-term allogenic T cell unresponsiveness in vitro. ILT2/CD85j is the only CD4[+] T cell receptor for HLA-G1 detected so far. Another HLA-G receptor may be expressed, but could not yet been identified.[26]

Another, maybe even more important HLA-G lymphocyte interaction is with CD8[+] T cells. Exposure of soluble HLA-G1 to activated, alloreactive (anti-paternal) CD8[+] T cells triggers the surface expression and secretion of the pro-apoptotic Fas-ligant, resulting in apoptosis of the activated T cells via the Fas/FasL pro-apoptotic pathway.[16,20,26,27,31]

In vitro studies demonstrated that FasL mRNA concentrations are eight times greater in cells incubated with sHLA molecules compared to control cells and the possibility of blocking the apoptosis by pre-incubating with amongst others anti-Fas m-antibody ZB4.[27,31]

The soluble form of HLA-G has been detected in amniotic fluid but also in low concentration in the sera of pregnant women, potentially to induce apoptosis of anti-paternal CD8[+] T cells not only at the site of placentation, but throughout the whole body. This assumption is further supported by the observation of higher levels of soluble HLA-G in women with male, compared to female offspring.[14,16]

Another mechanism to induce tolerance to fetal antigens beside the induction of apoptosis in CD8[+] T lymphocytes is the inhibition or reduction of their cytotoxic activity. The soluble HLA-G5 and the expression of the membrane-bound counterpart HLA-G1 can protect target cells from lyses by antigen-specific cytotoxic T cells. ILT2 directly compete with CD8 for binding to MHCs, whereas ILT2 has a higher binding affinity. This may effectively block CD8 binding at a cell-cell interface. Furthermore are ILT2 and TCR co-localized at the immunological synapse between T cells and APCs that express ILT ligands.

Here ILT2 could negatively influence the cytotoxicity of CD8[+] T cells not only by blocking the ligand binding of CD8 but also by recruiting the immunoreceptor tyrosine-based inhibitory receptor motifs to the vicinity of the TCR.[16,21]

6.2.2 B Cell Interactions

During pregnancies, mothers produce higher levels of antibodies due to the production of placental non-apoptosis-inducing TNF superfamily ligands, amongst others B cell-activating factor belonging to the TNF family (BAFF) and a proliferation-inducing factor (APRIL).[32] This mechanism ensures elevated host defense against pathogens and the transfer of protective antibodies to the fetus. In pregnant women it has been found that the production of antibodies against placental HLA-G barely occurs, what leads to the suggestion of a HLA-G-B lymphocyte crosstalk. In ninety-one per cent of all mothers, as well as all women who have never been pregnant and all men, there is no evidence of antibodies against HLA-G in the sera, measured by ELISA and immunoblotting. But still the nine per cent of women generating anti-HLA-G during their pregnancies show no difference in pregnancy-success compared to non-anti-HLA-G women. Besides T-lymphocytes and APCs, also B-lymphocytes express the ILT2 inhibitory receptors. Activation of B cell ILT2 receptors by circulating HLA-G5 or HLA-G6 could be one possible route to achieve this tolerance but still needs to be proven.

The activation of ILT2 receptors on Th cells could be the other possibility whereas APCs are driven into a B-lymphocyte-inhibiting, immunosuppressive profile. Th cells are abundant at the site of maternal-fetal interface where HLA-Gs are prominent.[16]

6.2.3 Monocyte Interactions

Monocytes are multifunctional lymphocytes giving rise to two populations, dendritic cells and macrophages, at the side of invasive cytotrophoblast cells, uterine glandular epithelium and the uterine blood vessels. One can distinguish between three different subgroups in the pregnant endometrium: CD14[+] macrophages, CD83[+] mature dendritic cells and CD83[-] immature macrophages/dendritic cells.[16] Decidual macrophages, which are activated in the pregnant uterus, have an immunosuppressive profile, producing prostaglandin E2 (PGE2) that acts in an autocrine manner to suppress its own activation and also in a paracrine way to inhibit alloactive T cells.[16,28] Furthermore they produce anti-inflammatory cytokines like IL-10 and transforming growth factor (TGF)-ß1.

Other markers of an immunosuppressive profile are B7-H1, ILT3, DC-SIGN, MS-1 and factor 13. A nearly similar DC-SIGN production is achieved by viral and bacterial pathogens followed by an alteration in cytokine production, leading to a benefit in pathogen survival.[16]

Mononuclear phagocytes as well as decidual macrophages, both express mainly ILT2 but also ILT4. Their mRNA could be found in decidual first-trimester macrophages due to RT-PCR measurements. Furthermore the proteins of ILT2 and ILT4 were detected by antibody labeling and flow cytometry, whereas CD163 was the marker for macrophages.[28]

These receptors are described for HLA-G binding, supporting the idea that this receptor-ligand binding might be the main stimulus for a change in gene expression. TGF-ß1 stimulates the formation of Treg subpopulation and IL-10 a TH-2 dominant condition, as mentioned earlier.[2][16][20] Furthermore HLA-G5 and HLA-G6 reduce CD8 mRNA and proteins in blood mononuclear cells that were activated by INFγ.[2]

7. Discussion and Conclusion

Placental trophoblast cells secrete immunosupressants like progesterone and also cytokines to create a side where cells of the innate immune system are abundant.[2] These cells are primarily CD56 [bright] Natural Killer cells and macrophages, whereas little cells of the acquired immune system are present, mainly T-lymphocytes.[2,3,6,7,9]

A normal immune response against foreign antigens, in case of the fetus, against paternal antigens, is mediated by cytotoxic T cells that recognize these antigens due to MHC class I presentation. Placental trophoblast cells of the placental villi do not at all express MHC class I antigens. The deeply invasive extravillous cytotrophoblast express only HLA-C and the non-classical class Ib HLA-E and HLA-G.[6,7,14] The MHC class I profile on cell surfaces is ´checked` by NK cells that circulate through the periphery, whereas a down-regulation or the absence of MHC class I molecules is recognized by NKs and seen as a pathologic cell-state. These cells are killed by NK cell mediated cytolyses.[18,19]

Concluding, the most important interaction at the side of trophoblast invasion is with NK cells and T cells.

The uNK cell receptor CD94/NKG2A complex is stimulated by HLA-E binding that is expressed by trophoblast cells. This receptor is coupled to intracellular immunoreceptor tyrosine based inhibition motifs that induce an inhibitory signal transduction cascade, inhibiting their cytolytic activity.[7,9] The HLA-G leading sequence seems to stimulate this signal positively when additively bound in the HLA-E binding groove.[6,9,20] A nearly similar effect is achieved by the binding of HLA-C to the KIR2/3DL receptor, only expressed by the uterine NK subpopulation, also leading to an inhibitory signal transduction.[9,19] Another interaction is mediated by HLA-G1 and ILT-2. This interaction results in a strong NK cell inhibition of all NK cells.[21] So this unique interaction of ligands, expressed by placental trophoblast cells and uNK cell receptors prevents NK cell mediated killing of placental cells.

Actually the most important molecule in fetal immune tolerance achievement is HLA-G. Monocytes infected with HLA-G1 secrete cytokines like TGF-ß1 and IL-10 that drives T cell into an immunosuppressive TH-2 cytokine producing lymphocyte.[2,16,20] These cells further reduce the maturation of CD8[+] T cells into a cytotoxic T cells appearance.[26] Another maybe even more important interaction with T cells is the direct contact of activated, alloreactive (anti-paternal) CD8[+] T cells with soluble HLA-G1.

HLA-G1 stimulates the expression and secretion of the pro-apoptotic Fas-ligant, resulting in a Fas/FasL binding and induction of an apoptotic pathway, which reduces the number of CD8$^+$ T cells, reactive for paternal antigens in the periphery.[16,20,26,27,31]

Recapitulating it can be said that a special MHC expression profile of placental trophoblast cells as well as the secretion of hormones and cytokines protect the fetus across the placenta from being rejected by the maternal immune system. HLA-C, HLA-E and particularly HLA-G can be seen as the ´survival-molecules` of placental cells against NK cells and activated, anti-paternal cytotoxic T lymphocytes.

Still a great problem is to extrapolate the in vitro assays to the in vivo situation at the side of implantation. Reasons are practical and ethnical difficulties in generating clones of human placental and decidual cells. Further research in the field of placental-uterine crosstalk bears deep insights in molecular mechanisms of immunology multidisciplinary necessary.

A high number of transferred in vitro fertilization (IVF) embryos, approximate 70 per cent, fail to implant, whereas only about 14 per cent of these embryos will succeed pregnancy.[29] The development of maternal as well embryonic makers could prevent that high number of failure.

Studies showed that HLA-G is also a molecule that is expressed by tumor cells to circumvent a host immune response.[20] That makes HLA-G a target of interest in oncology and cancer research. Furthermore could just that feature of cancer cells be a new improvement in tissue and organ transplantations, to facilitate acceptance of implanted allografts.

Interactions between HLA and maternal immune cells		
Interactions	Results	Literature
NK cell		
CD94/NKG2 – HLA-E	Net inhibitory signal	A Moffett-King [6] A King at al. [9] A Moffett at al. [7]
KIR – HLA-C	Net inhibitory signal	A King at al. [9] S Rajagopalan at al. [19]
ILT2 – HLAG1	Inhibitory signal on peripheral NKs	A King at al. [9] M Shiroishi at al. [21]
CD4+ T cell		
ILT2 – HLA-G	Th2 immunosuppressive profile	JS Hunt at al. [16] (in vitro studies) K Kapasi at al. [25] (in vitro studies) I Noci at al. [29] (in vitro studies) T Kanai at al. [30] (in vitro studies)
CD8+ T cell		
HLA-G exposure	Apoptosis induction in alloreactive cells	JS Hunt at al. [16] (in vitro studies) JS Hunt at al. [20] (in vitro studies) J LeMaoult at al. [26] S Fournel at al. [27] P Contini at al. [31]
ILT2 - HLA-G	Reduced cytotoxicity	JS Hunt at al. [16] (in vitro studies) M Shiroishi at al. [21]
Monocytes		
ILT2/4 – HLA-G	Production of anti-inflammatory cytokines Stimulation of Th2 conditions	JS Hunt at al. [2] JS Hunt at al. [16] (in vitro studies) JS Hunt at al. [20] (in vitro studies)

Table 2: Literature about interactions between HLAs and maternal cells.

8. References

1: Entfällt

2: Hunt JS. Stranger in a strange land. Immunol Rev. 2006 Oct;213:36-47. Review.

3: Parham P. NK cells and trophoblasts: partners in pregnancy. J Exp Med. 2004 Oct 18;200(8):951-5. Review

4: Ji Q, Luo ZX, Yuan CX, Wible JR, Zhang JP, Georgi JA. The earliest known eutherian mammal. Nature. 2002 Apr 25;416(6883):816-22.

5: Rama S, Rao AJ. Regulation of growth and function of the human placenta. Mol Cell Biochem. 2003 Nov;253(1-2):263-8. Review.

6: Moffett-King A.Natural killer cells and pregnancy. Nat Rev Immunol. 2002 Sep;2(9):656-63. Review.

7: Moffett A, Loke C. Immunology of placentation in eutherian mammals. Nat Rev Immunol. 2006 Aug;6(8):584-94. Review.

8: Gude NM, Roberts CT, Kalionis B, King RG. Growth and function of the normal human placenta. Thromb Res. 2004;114(5-6):397-407. Review.

9: King A, Hiby SE, Gardner L, Joseph S, Bowen JM, Verma S, Burrows TD, Loke YW. Recognition of trophoblast HLA class I molecules by decidual NK cell receptors--a review. Placenta. 2000 Mar-Apr;21 Suppl A:S81-5. Review.

10: Scott F. Gilbert. Developmental Biology, Eighth Edition, 2006 Palgrave Macmillan, 11: 348

11: William J. Larsen. Human Embryology, Third Edition, 2001 Churchill Livingstone, 1: 18-22

12: Scott F. Gilbert. Developmental Biology, Eighth Edition, 2006 Palgrave Macmillan, 11: 348-355

13: Chaddha V, Viero S, Huppertz B, Kingdom J. Developmental biology of the placenta and the origins of placental insufficiency. Semin Fetal Neonatal Med. 2004 Oct;9(5):357-69. Review.

14: Huddleston H, Schust DJ. Immune interactions at the maternal-fetal interface: a focus on antigen presentation. Am J Reprod Immunol. 2004 Apr;51(4):283-9. Review.

15: Blois S, Tometten M, Kandil J, Hagen E, Klapp BF, Margni RA, Arck PC. Intercellular adhesion molecule-1/LFA-1 cross talk is a proximate mediator capable of disrupting immune integration and tolerance mechanism at the feto-maternal interface in murine pregnancies. J Immunol. 2005 Feb 15;174(4):1820-9.

16: Hunt JS, Petroff MG, McIntire RH, Ober C. HLA-G and immune tolerance in pregnancy. FASEB J. 2005 May;19(7):681-93. Review.

17: Roderick Neirn, Matthew Helbert. Immunology for medical students, 2002 Mosby, 15: 129-130

18: Vosshenrich CA, Samson-Villeger SI, Di Santo JP. Distinguishing features of developing natural killer cells. Curr Opin Immunol. 2005 Apr;17(2):151-8. Review.

19: Rajagopalan S, Bryceson YT, Kuppusamy SP, Geraghty DE, van der Meer A, Joosten I, Long EO. Activation of NK cells by an endocytosed receptor for soluble HLA-G. PLoS Biol. 2006 Jan;4(1):e9.

20: Hunt JS, Morales PJ, Pace JL, Fazleabas AT, Langat DK. A commentary on gestational programming and functions of HLA-G in pregnancy. Placenta. 2007 Apr;28 Suppl A:S57-63. Epub 2007 Mar 9.

21: Shiroishi M, Tsumoto K, Amano K, Shirakihara Y, Colonna M, Braud VM at al., Human inhibitory receptors Ig-like transcript 2 (ILT2) and ILT4 compete with CD8 for MHC class I binding and bind preferentially to HLA-G. Proc Natl Acad Sci U S A. 2003 Jul 22;100(15):8856-61.

22: Roche Medizin Lexikon online, HLA System:
http://www.tkonline.de/rochelexikon/ro15000/r16259.000.html

23: Roderick Neirn, Matthew Helbert. Immunology for medical students, 2002 Mosby, 21: 183

24: King A, Burrows TD, Hiby SE, Bowen JM, Joseph S, Verma S, Lim PB, Gardner L, Le Bouteiller P, Ziegler A, Uchanska-Ziegler B, Loke YW. Surface expression of HLA-C antigen by human extravillous trophoblast. Placenta. 2000 May;21(4):376-87.

25: Kapasi K, Albert SE, Yie S, Zavazava N, Librach CL. HLA-G has a concentration-dependent effect on the generation of an allo-CTL response. Immunology. 2000 Oct;101(2):191-200.

26: LeMaoult J, Krawice-Radanne I, Dausset J, Carosella ED. HLA-G1-expressing antigen-presenting cells induce immunosuppressive CD4+ T cells. Proc Natl Acad Sci U S A. 2004 May 4;101(18):7064-9.

27: Fournel S, Aguerre-Girr M, Huc X, Lenfant F, Alam A, Toubert A, Bensussan A, Le Bouteiller P. Cutting edge: soluble HLA-G1 triggers CD95/CD95 ligand-mediated apoptosis in activated CD8+ cells by interacting with CD8. J Immunol. 2000 Jun 15;164(12):6100-4.

28: Petroff MG, Sedlmayr P, Azzola D, Hunt JS. Decidual macrophages are potentially susceptible to inhibition by class Ia and class Ib HLA molecules. J Reprod Immunol. 2002 Jul-Aug;56(1-2):3-17.

29: Noci I, Fuzzi B, Rizzo R, Melchiorri L, Criscuoli L, Dabizzi S, Biagiotti R, Pellegrini S, Menicucci A, Baricordi OR. Embryonic soluble HLA-G as a marker of developmental potential in embryos. Hum Reprod. 2005 Jan;20(1):138-46. Epub 2004 Oct 21.

30: Kanai T, Fujii T, Kozuma S, Yamashita T, Miki A, Kikuchi A, Taketani Y. Soluble HLA-G influences the release of cytokines from allogeneic peripheral blood mononuclear cells in culture. Mol Hum Reprod. 2001 Feb;7(2):195-200

31: Contini P, Ghio M, Poggi A, Filaci G, Indiveri F, Ferrone S, Puppo F. Soluble HLA-A,-B,-C and -G molecules induce apoptosis in T and NK CD8+ cells and inhibit cytotoxic T cell activity through CD8 ligation. Eur J Immunol. 2003 Jan;33(1):125-34.

32: Phillips TA, Ni J, Hunt JS. Cell-specific expression of B lymphocyte (APRIL, BLyS)- and Th2 (CD30L/CD153)-promoting tumor necrosis factor superfamily ligands in human placentas. J Leukoc Biol. 2003 Jul;74(1):81-7.

33: Colucci F, Caligiuri MA, Di Santo JP. What does it take to make a natural killer? Nat Rev Immunol. 2003 May;3(5):413-25. Review.